101 Female Health Secrets

every woman must know

from the editors of **PREVENTION**® Magazine Health Books

Copyright 1996 by Roda   D1279935   ̷

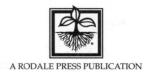

A RODALE PRESS PUBLICATION

Editorial/design manager: Terry Rush-Mamenko, Ph.D.
Project editors: Diane K. Gilroy, Beth W. Orenstein, and Beth Gehman
Copy editor: Christine Brandt Little
Cover designer: Debbie Buhosky
Book designer: Kathi L. Shoemaker
Illustrator: Susan Rosenberger

CONTENTS

Taking charge of your own health can make the difference between a long and vigorous life and a short one plagued with problems you shouldn't even have to think about until you're 90. Taking charge is easier than you think. Basically, you must do two things—follow a screening schedule based on your personal risk factors and adopt proven preventive measures. Screenings are important because early detection often means you have more treatment options and a better chance of a full recovery. Making healthy lifestyle changes, such as following a low-fat diet, exercising, and quitting smoking, can prevent many health problems from ever developing.

This book will show you how to take charge of your health by helping you plan your screening schedule and prevent your most common health concerns. We've even provided a sample medical log to help you keep track of your doctors, screening schedule, and other health needs.

So use this book and take charge of your health.

5

CHAPTER 1
CHOOSING DR. RIGHT

Getting a checkup seems simple enough, but when you start looking for a doctor, it can quickly start to resemble the quest for the Holy Grail. Who's qualified? What should you, as a smart consumer, be looking for?

"Basically, anyone who holds himself out by training and practice as a primary care physician should be fully qualified to take care of checkups for normal, healthy adults," says Douglas Kamerow, M.D., director of the Clinical Preventive Services Staff for the Office of Disease Prevention and Health Promotion in the U.S. Public Health Service. "But, in my opinion, there are really only two groups that are qualified by their training to do so: general internists and family physicians."

Some experts in women's health, however, would narrow the list even more and add a few provisos. "My number-one choice would be a general internist," says Lila Wallis, M.D., clinical professor of medicine at Cornell University Medical College, former president of the American Medical Women's Association (AMWA), and founder of the National Council of Women's Health in New York City. "And not just any general internist, but one who has had special training in office gynecology and the psychological needs of female patients."

According to Dr. Wallis, a family practitioner would do if a general internist was not available. "The only reason he or she wouldn't be my first choice is that the family practitioner has to learn so much more about children that it could dilute the amount of time spent keeping abreast of women's health developments."

While many women make gynecologists their first choice, they actually come in third as far as Dr. Wallis is concerned. "While general internists and family practitioners already have a firm knowledge of the rest of the body, gynecologists specialize specifically in women's sexual organs and reproductive tract," she notes. "This gives them far more to learn than the other two to become a primary care physician."

Specialization is not something you want to overlook, adds Dr. Wallis. "Many internists have areas of specialization such as cardiology or hematology. But you want to be careful that they aren't neglecting continuing education courses in women's health issues to the advantage of their other interest."

HOW OFTEN SHOULD YOU GO?

Back in 1922 the American Medical Association (AMA) first endorsed the annual examination of healthy people, and for many years it was standard practice. "It was only in 1983 that the AMA withdrew support for this concept," says Douglas Kamerow, M.D., director of the Clinical Preventive Services Staff for the Office of Disease Prevention and Health Promotion in the U.S. Public Health Service.

In this brave new world of checkups, the current medical wisdom is that for healthy people, a more tailored program of preventive services can be effective. In layman's terms, this means fewer checkups will do just as well as the time-honored annual physical.

If you have no serious ailments that need monitoring, most experts advise that you touch base with your primary care physician every three to five years from age 30 to 39, every two to three years from age 40 to 49, and past age 50, every year.

But, adds Dr. Kamerow, an annual Pap smear is still recommended regardless of your age if you have shown any potential signs of trouble in the cervix or if you have multiple sex partners.

Especially for Women

One big clue to whether a physician is informed about women's health is if she does careful breast and pelvic exams during the annual physical.

Another clue is whether the physician asks about issues that are particularly important to women at each stage of life. For example, Dr. Wallis says, young women should be asked about body image, eating disorders, and calcium intake. For women in the middle years, it's particularly important to ask about multiple stressors, which could stem from caring for elders and children, as well as sleep and weight changes, and coping with menopause. For seniors, bone health, social contacts, and abuse by spouse or by caregivers are examples of issues to which physicians should be sensitive.

Under Dr. Wallis's supervision, the AMWA developed a comprehensive women's health curriculum that it offers to interested physicians.

Women's health, they feel, combines internal medicine, obstetrics and gynecology, family practice, and psychiatry. But, Dr. Wallis adds, re-educating doctors won't do the whole job.

"We'll need to teach women how to be responsible partners in their health care," says Dr. Wallis. "With health reforms on the horizon, physicians may spend even less time with each patient. So women need to be even more assertive."

Preparing for Your Checkup

Miss Marple may have been able to get to the truth based on the merest of clues, but your doctor needs solid information. The best way to provide that information is to do a bit of homework before your visit.

Keep a food log. When it comes to health habits, the murkiest information tends to surround diet. How often do you really notice what you eat throughout the day: that mid-morning candy bar, a bag of chips in the car. It all adds up, but it's easily forgettable when making a report on your eating habits to your doctor. What in reality is not the healthiest of eating habits can suddenly become squeaky clean in the doctor's office.

"If you know you're going in for a checkup and plan on discussing diet, it's not a bad idea to keep a precise food log for a week beforehand," suggests Dr. Kamerow. "Don't change your eating habits, just keep track of them. It's the little forgettable things like snacks that add up to a lot of dietary fat, and it's these things that you'll need to focus on when talking to your doctor."

9

Climb your family tree. Coming up with a complete family history of illnesses also will require a little attention and, depending on what you discover, may affect the types of tests you'll need. "People with a family history of certain health problems may be at greater risk of developing them, and it's reasonable to screen these people more regularly or earlier for these diseases," says Dr. Kamerow.

While there may well be hundreds of diseases that can be passed along genetically, there are, in fact, only a few that you really need to be concerned with. "Breast cancer is a primary concern," says Dr. Kamerow. "The U.S. Preventive Services Task Force does not recommend mammograms before the age of 50. But one may want to make an exception for women who are at high risk by evidence that their mother or sister had it, especially if the cancer was pre-menopausal."

Osteoporosis is another concern for women. "A family history of osteoporosis might predispose me to suggest a bone mineral density study at menopause, which I might not normally use routinely," says Dr. Wallis. A family history of heart disease or any cancer, including ovarian, colon, breast, uterine, and pancreatic, also should be discussed with your doctor.

Prepare your files. You'll want to make sure your doctor has records from any other physicians you may have visited. You'll also want to inform her of any medications you are taking and any problems that you feel you may be experiencing because of them. You also may want to prepare a list of current health complaints complete with symptoms and dates if possible.

Getting the Most from Your Checkup

You've picked the doc, done your homework, and now you're cooling your heels in the waiting room listening to a Muzak version of "Eleanor Rigby." What lies in wait for you beyond the smiling nurse? Or, more to the point, what should happen in the examination room to make for a perfect checkup?

"One of the most important components of the physical is a breast examination," says JoAnn E. Manson, M.D., co-principal investigator of the cardiovascular component of the Nurses' Health Study, associate professor of medicine at Harvard Medical School, and co-director of women's health at Brigham and Women's Hospital, both in Boston. "After that and, of course, a pelvic exam and Pap smear, there is a whole list of options that can be performed, some more important than others."

Dr. Manson strongly suggests that your doctor perform the following:

- Measure your blood pressure, weight, and height.
- Inspect your tongue and gums for any signs of oral cancer or need for dental care.
- Check the artery in your neck for pulse and listen for bruits—abnormal sounds that can indicate a clogged artery.
- Inspect the neck area for thyroid size and nodules for possible signs of cancer.
- Examine your skin, especially in sun-exposed areas, for any signs of skin cancer.
- Listen to your chest for heart sounds and lung congestion, crackles, or wheezes.

"In some people, especially those who are young and healthy, it may be less important to check the liver, kidneys, spleen, and reflexes and test for signs of nerve damage," says Dr. Manson. "The need for many of these tests depends on age, prior medical history, and risk factors. So not all women should expect to have all these tests performed at every checkup."

What else might you expect?

"It's also not a bad idea to do a nonfasting total blood cholesterol screening, and this is especially needed if there is a history of heart disease in the family," says Dr. Kamerow.

Pap smears are also standard issue. Regular Pap smears are especially important for sexually active women outside of a monogamous relationship, because many physicians feel that the human papilloma virus, a sexually transmitted disease, is a major cause of cervical cancer. If your sexual activity is not directed toward only one person, Dr. Kamerow suggests that you get routine screenings for other sexually transmitted diseases, such as chlamydia, as well.

Taking the Doctor's Advice Home

Take a deep breath and relax. The poking and prodding are behind you. Now it's time to direct the hard light of science onto your lifestyle. "Outside of the few tests and shots you should get, the most important thing that can be done at a checkup is to team up with your doctor and take stock of your health habits," states Dr. Kamerow. The big four topics of discussion should be exercise, diet, sexual practices, and vices such as smoking and drinking, he says. "Poor habits in these areas contribute mightily to the leading causes of disease and death in this country, and yet they are the very things we cannot test or fix with medicine."

If you smoke, talk to your doctor about ways to quit. The same goes for "recreational" drugs, alcohol abuse, and excessive use of medications, such as sedatives and diet pills. If you are prone to adventurous sex, have a sobering conversation on safe sex as well as the potential dangers involved in bed hopping. Diet? Haul out that food diary and go over it in detail. As for exercise, ask your doctor for tips to incorporate more physical activity into your life.

Also, it's a good idea to discuss your screening schedule with your primary care physician at least once a year. Changes in screening guidelines or in your personal risk factors might suggest that your screening schedule needs updating. Says Janet Rose Osuch, M.D., of the AMWA, "Most doctors are not going to get upset by a gentle reminder to talk about medical screening tests—they're going to be grateful. The patient is not just saying, 'Do you think I need a mammogram?' but also, 'I'm willing to go get one, and I'm asking for your expert advice.'"

Whenever you have a test, it's a good idea to write down the results. Call your doctor after each test to discuss it. That practice has the added advantage of forcing the doctor to look at your test results.

Don't worry about taking up too much of your doctor's time. "The most important thing that goes on at a checkup is the counseling and the activity that the patient then does because of that counseling," says Dr. Kamerow. "Doctors are beginning to realize that the most healing thing they can do is provide information and motivation."

11

CHAPTER 2
THE TOP 15 TESTS FOR WOMEN

Which medical screening tests should you have regularly? Each woman's needs are different, based on her age, genetics, medical history, and lifestyle. Use the following information to help you and your physician determine a screening schedule that's best for you. Keep in mind that these are general guidelines for women, approved by AMWA physicians. Admittedly, some may differ slightly from those recommended by other professional associations. Nevertheless, the list is a good starting point for discussions with your physician. We've included checkboxes to help you personalize the information.

12 Heart Health

Heart disease is the leading cause of death among American women, striking down half a million each year. If you follow the guidelines below, symptoms of heart disease can be detected early and possibly reversed by lifestyle measures and/or medication.

1. **Blood pressure check.** A measurement of blood pressure taken with an inflatable cuff, known as a sphygmomanometer.
   - ☐ Once every year if you are age 19 to 40 with no heart disease risk factors and are not taking oral contraceptives.
   - ☐ Twice or more every year if you are older than 40; take oral contraceptives; have borderline high blood pressure (140/90 or greater); have a personal history of high blood pressure or heart disease; are on blood pressure medication; have a family history of high blood pressure and/or heart disease; smoke; are very overweight; regularly take over-the-counter non-steroidal anti-inflammatory medications (analgesics); or for other reasons, at a physician's recommendation.

NOTE: A healthy blood-pressure reading should be less than 140 systolic over less than 90 diastolic.

2. **Blood cholesterol test.** A small blood sample is analyzed at the doctor's office or in a laboratory, after a 12-hour fast, because triglycerides are very sensitive to diet. This would include total cholesterol plus high-density lipoprotein (HDL) and low-density lipoprotein (LDL) ratios in addition to your triglyceride level.

☐ Once every year at any age if you are in good health. "Even screening in childhood may be of benefit and should be continued lifelong," says AMWA cardiologist Debra Judelson, M.D.

☐ Twice or more every year if you have recently gained a great deal of weight; have become sedentary; have become ill; have borderline high cholesterol (about 200 to 240); have high cholesterol (above 240); are on cholesterol-lowering medication; have diabetes or kidney disease; have HDL (good cholesterol) levels below 35; have undergone removal of the ovaries; have recently undergone menopause; have heart disease or symptoms of heart disease; or for other reasons, at a physician's recommendation.

NOTE: Healthy readings for women should be approximately 160 for total cholesterol, 50 or higher for HDL, below 120 for LDL, and below 110 for triglycerides.

3. **Exercise stress test.** Requires exercise on a treadmill while the heart is monitored externally.

☐ One screening test, possibly followed by repeated tests every two to five years if you are older than age 40; are older than age 30 and have strong risk factors for heart disease, such as high blood pressure, diabetes, significant obesity, smoking, family history of heart disease; have had your ovaries removed; have high cholesterol; have symptoms of heart disease; or for other reasons, at a physician's recommendation.

NOTE: For 40 percent of women who take the exercise stress test, the result is a false-positive—in other words, it indicates problems when there are none. If your test findings are abnormal, your physician may refer you for more sophisticated tests, like a stress echocardiogram, involving exercise and ultrasound, or a nuclear medicine test, involving an injection of radioactive material. If you are at a high risk for heart disease, your physician may skip the exercise stress test and go directly to the more sensitive tests.

Breast Care

Some 180,000 women in the United States were diagnosed with breast cancer in 1994; as many as 46,000 of those women died. But AMWA experts say that if all women followed the guidelines below, a third of breast cancer deaths could be avoided.

4. **Breast self-examination (BSE).** The careful self-palpation of each breast, preferably the week after a woman's monthly menstrual period, to check for any unusual lumps or masses.

☐ Once every month if you are older than age 16. By that age, most women's breasts are fully developed, and doctors say it's best to learn BSE when you're young, so it becomes a lifelong habit.

NOTE: To learn how to perform BSE, see pages 27 to 29, ask your physician for guidance, or check with your community hospital, woman's health clinic, or local American Cancer Society office for classes.

5. **Breast examination by a qualified health professional.** Visual examination and careful palpation of the breasts and underarms by a qualified physician or health professional. The practitioner should examine your breasts while you are sitting up and lying down, too.

☐ Once every two to three years if you are age 16 to 39 and have no risk factors for or symptoms of breast cancer.

☐ Once every year or more frequently if you are older than age 40; have lumpy breasts that are difficult to self-examine; do not perform monthly breast self-examinations; have risk factors for breast cancer, such as a family history of the disease, no children before age 30, breast biopsies that show atypical epithelial hyperplasia, or a personal history of breast cancer; or for other reasons at a doctor's recommendation.

6. **Mammography.** Low-dose breast x-ray. The apparatus compresses the breast firmly between two plates, which may cause discomfort. Usually two or three views per breast are required for a complete screening.

☐ One baseline test, followed by additional tests every one to two years if you are age 40 to 49 and don't have risk factors for or symptoms of breast cancer.

☐ Once every year if you are age 50 or older; have risk factors for breast cancer (see #5 above) regardless of your age; or at a doctor's recommendation.

NOTE: Most physicians recommend women schedule their mammogram for the week after their menstrual period, to minimize discomfort.

There is controversy over whether most women younger than age 50 need regular mammograms. Some studies suggest that mammography in younger women doesn't significantly reduce death rates. However, Dr. Osuch points out, even if that unproven contention is true, early detection through mammography does give younger women more treatment options, like breast-saving lumpectomy. Until there's more data, the AMWA says it's still a good idea for women to begin getting regular mammograms at age 40.

14

Gynecological Care

Women are susceptible to a wide range of gynecological problems, ranging from vaginal infections and uterine fibroids to cervical abnormalities and ovarian growths. That's why careful annual pelvic examinations, along with the screening tests described here, are an essential part of a woman's annual physical exam. With early detection, most gynecological problems can be treated successfully.

7. Pelvic examination. A manual examination of the vaginal area by a qualified health professional to check for any abnormalities of the uterus and ovaries. Usually, the doctor places—carefully and gently—two gloved fingers in the vagina while the other hand presses firmly on top of the abdomen.
☐ Once every year if you are older than age 18.

8. Pap test. After inserting a speculum into the vagina and opening it to reveal the cervix, the doctor scrapes cells from the cervix and the cervical canal and smears them on a slide. The sample is sent to a laboratory, which examines it for signs of cervical cancer.
☐ Once every year if you are older than age 18.

NOTE: Cervical cancer has been linked to certain strains of the human papilloma virus. This virus can be transmitted through sexual intercourse. But any woman can develop cervical cancer at any age, regardless of sexual activity. Seniors still need to be tested regularly, even if they don't have a partner. This is true even after a hysterectomy if the cervix is left intact. (If your cervix has been removed, you still need Pap smears. Check with your doctor to see how often.)

9. Transvaginal ultrasound. An ultrasonic probe is inserted into the vagina, transmitting images of the uterus and ovaries to a monitoring screen. It's sometimes used as a screening tool to detect changes in the ovaries and the lining of the uterus that might suggest cancer.
☐ One screening test, possibly followed by others at the recommendation of a physician if you are at or past menopause and may be at risk for endometrial cancer. May also be used for women of any age who have a strong family history (in your immediate family—mother, sister, or daughter) or other significant risk factors for ovarian cancer.

10. Endometrial tissue sample. A thin instrument is inserted through the vagina and cervical opening to remove a tiny tissue sample from the lining of the uterus. Also called an endometrial biopsy or aspiration, the procedure can cause cramping.
☐ One screening test, possibly followed by others, at intervals recommended by a physician if you're past menopause and are considering or currently taking hormone-replacement therapy;

are taking tamoxifen; eat a very high-fat diet; have a history of infertility; have a history of not ovulating; are very overweight; have a family history of endometrial cancer; exhibit abnormal uterine bleeding; or if your doctor has recommended it for other reasons.

NOTE: To avoid damage to the uterus, endometrial sampling should be performed by an experienced physician.

Colon Cancer Prevention

Colon cancer is the third leading cancer among women, after breast and lung cancer. More women are affected by colon cancer annually (56,000) than are men (53,000). But the following screening recommendations could help nip those cancers in the bud. These tests can help detect precancerous changes and early cancer, which usually can be treated easily.

11. **Digital-rectal exam.** With a gloved finger, a physician feels inside the rectum for abnormalities.
    - ☐ Once every year if you are age 40 or older.

12. **Fecal occult blood test.** A stool sample is usually brought to a physician's office, hospital, or clinic for analysis. (The stool sample also can be obtained in the doctor's office.) The test seeks blood as a possible symptom of colorectal cancer.
    - ☐ Once every year if you're age 50 or older.

NOTE: The fecal occult blood test has been criticized because of its high rate of false positives (wrongly indicating a possibility of cancer) and false negatives (missing the cancer when it's really there). But it's important to remember that, while a positive result may not mean cancer, it can indicate ulcers, hemorrhoids, or other problems. For a definitive diagnosis of colorectal cancer, more sophisticated tests are required (such as sigmoidoscopy, discussed below).

13. **Sigmoidoscopy.** A thin, hollow, lighted tube is inserted into the rectum and lower part of the colon to look for precancerous polyps and remove them before a cancer develops. Flexible sigmoidoscopes are preferred because they cause less discomfort than rigid scopes.
    - ☐ Once every three to five years if you are age 50 or older and have no colorectal cancer risk factors or symptoms.
    - ☐ More than once every three years, at the discretion of the physician, if you have a personal history of colon polyps, chronic inflammatory bowel disease, or colorectal cancer; a family history of colon polyps or colorectal cancer (especially if a member of your immediate family—parent, sibling, or child—developed colon cancer before age 50); symptoms of colorectal cancer (such as

diarrhea, constipation, or both, blood in the stools, very narrow stools, unexplained weight loss, or frequent gas pains and general stomach discomfort); a feeling that the bowel does not empty completely; a history of breast, endometrial, or ovarian cancer; or if your physician has recommended it for other reasons.

Bone Health

One in two women will develop fractures from osteoporosis in her lifetime, and complications of hip fractures account for 50,000 deaths every year. "There's no reason we can't prevent most hip fractures and deaths from osteoporosis if we combine early detection and treatment," says AMWA osteoporosis expert Sydney Bonnick, M.D.

14. **Bone scan.** Bone scans are performed by machines that use low-dose radiation. You sit or lie on a table with the machine's energy sources above and/or below you. Depending on the technology, this painless procedure may take 5 to 30 minutes.

☐ One baseline screening just before menopause or very early in menopause; one more test a year to 18 months after menopause. In some cases, more follow-up tests may be required. Older or younger women also may require testing, depending on their risk factors for osteoporosis (family history, steroid use, low-calcium diet, or sedentary lifestyle) or if their physicians have recommended it.

NOTE: A bone scan can show women who are approaching menopause whether they are at risk for osteoporosis and should take estrogen or other medication (such as salmon calcitonin or etidronate) to prevent further bone weakening. It also provides a baseline measurement, so that a year after menopause, a repeat scan can determine whether you have lost too much bone and need to begin medication or adjust your current dosage.

Several different technologies are available for measuring bone density, including dual energy x-ray absorptiometry, dual photon absorptiometry, single photon absorptiometry, quantitative computed tomography, and radiographic absorptiometry. All of the techniques are capable of detecting low bone mass and diagnosing osteoporosis, according to Sandra C. Raymond, executive director of the National Osteoporosis Foundation. She points out that "some experts believe that for predicting fracture risk, the specific bone at risk for fracturing should be measured."

It's not always easy to find a facility for a bone density test. The National Osteoporosis Foundation suggests checking with a local academic health center, a major hospital, or the local branch of the AMA.

Even major medical centers may not perform tests accurately.

17

"It's a problem all of us recognize and are trying to improve," says Dr. Bonnick. In the meantime, ask the technician whether he or she has had several years of experience with bone scans. And make sure the physician will be reviewing the test and providing a written interpretation—don't settle for a computer printout-based diagnosis. Raymond emphasizes that "a bone mass measurement should be performed in the context of a total medical assessment by a qualified physician."

AIDS Prevention

There are many powerful reasons for women—and their partners—to be tested for human immunodeficiency virus (HIV). That's because transmission of the AIDS virus in the United States goes back to 1977.

15. HIV test. A blood sample is taken for analysis. If an anonymous test site analyzes the sample, results are returned in 10 to 14 days. Private physicians may return results sooner.

☐ One screening test with follow-up tests at least three to six months after last possible exposure to the virus, if you had a blood transfusion between 1977 and 1985; if you have had sexual intercourse since 1977 with any partner whose sexual, transfusion or drug use history since 1977 is uncertain; or if you have ever injected drugs with shared needles.

18

NOTE: For the vast majority of people, an HIV test at least three months after the last possible exposure indicates whether HIV is present. However, in very rare cases, the telltale antibodies to HIV don't show up in the blood until six months after the last exposure. We suggest taking a test at three months and continuing to abstain from sex or to practice safer sex (limiting activity to nonpenetration or careful and consistent use of condoms) until a test after six months from the last possible exposure.

Many people are reluctant to get an HIV test through their physicians because they are concerned about their anonymity. Fortunately, there are anonymous test sites in every state. They never take names, identifying clients only through a number. To locate these sites, call your state health department and ask for the HIV/AIDS department. Or call the Centers for Disease Control and Prevention's toll-free national AIDS hotline at (800) 342-AIDS. Spanish speakers can call (800) 344-SIDA.

The American Medical Women's Association (AMWA) is a national association of women physicians and medical students. Founded in 1915, AMWA works to promote women's health and the role of women in medicine.

CHAPTER 3
STAY HEALTHY TIPS

Some of the tips that follow may seem repetitive because they are. But preventive measures, such as a healthy diet, regular exercise, and not smoking, are key to heading off a number of common diseases and conditions among women. So think of it this way: While you're eating a low-fat diet and exercising for a healthy heart, you're also helping prevent cancer and osteoporosis.

Heart Health
Control Blood Pressure

Lots of prescription drugs help reduce high blood pressure. Diuretics flush excess fluids from the body. Beta-blockers reduce the heart rate and the heart's total output of blood. Vasodilators widen arteries and allow easier blood flow. Sympathetic nerve inhibitors also prevent blood vessels from constricting.

19

But drugs should be a last resort. They can cause fatigue and inhibit your sex life, among other problems. The trick is to avoid high blood pressure in the first place. The tips below will get you started. Even if you already have mild high blood pressure, following these suggestions could reduce your dependence on drugs and maybe even let you control things naturally.

Lighten up. If you're overweight, even moderate weight loss may help lower your blood pressure, says Marvin Moser, M.D., clinical professor of medicine at Yale University School of Medicine and senior advisor to the National High Blood Pressure Education Program. In some cases, he says, weight loss of 10 to 15 pounds may be enough to lower slightly elevated blood pressure to normal levels and help you avoid medication.

Move it. Exercise, combined with a low-fat diet, is the best way to lose weight and keep your arteries clog-free. Research shows that people who don't exercise are 35 to 50 percent more likely to develop high blood pressure. And the American College of Sports Medicine says that regular aerobic training can reduce systolic and diastolic blood pressure by as much as 10 points.

You don't have to be a marathon runner to reap the benefits, either. In fact, some studies have found that lower intensity workouts such as walking are as good or better at lowering blood pressure than running or other heavy-duty aerobic activities. Many experts recommend working out at least three times a week for 20 minutes a pop.

Shake it off. Remember that not everyone is sensitive to the effects of sodium. But until doctors can reliably tell who is and who isn't, it's a good idea to limit your intake. "It certainly isn't going to hurt anyone to cut down on salt and probably will be of real value if you're successful," says Robert DiBianco, M.D., director of cardiology research at the Washington Adventist Hospital in Takoma Park, Maryland.

Cut salt from your diet wherever you can. Most of us are eating about 2½ times more than we should. Swearing off the table shaker will have some effect. But research shows that three-fourths of all the salt we eat comes from processed foods such as cheese, soup, bread, baked goods, and snacks.

"You have to read labels," says Patrick Mulrow, M.D., chairman of the Department of Medicine at the Medical College of Ohio in Toledo and chairman of the American Heart Association's Council for High Blood Pressure Research. Check for sodium content and shoot for a daily total of about 2,400 milligrams. When shopping, look for labels that say "low sodium." That means they contain no more than 140 milligrams of sodium per serving. And spend some extra time in the produce aisle. Almost every fruit and vegetable is naturally low in sodium.

Be careful when you eat out, too. You'll be surprised how fast sodium can add up. A hamburger from your favorite fast food restaurant, for instance, may give you almost half a day's total.

Pile on the potassium. Studies have shown that eating 3,500 milligrams of potassium can help counteract sodium and keep blood volume—and blood pressure—down. And it's easy to get enough. A baked potato packs 838 milligrams of potassium all by itself, and one cup of spinach has 800 milligrams. Other potassium-packed foods include bananas, orange juice, corn, cabbage, and broccoli. But check with your doctor before taking potassium supplements. Too much potassium may aggravate kidney problems.

Meet your magnesium needs. Researchers seem to have found a link between low magnesium intake and high blood pressure. But just how much magnesium you need to combat high blood pressure remains unclear. For now, Dr. DiBianco says, your best bet is to get the Daily Value (DV) of about 280 milligrams.

Unfortunately, America's intake of magnesium has been dropping for a century, since we started processing foods and robbing them of their trace elements. Good sources of magnesium include nuts, spinach, lima beans, peas, and seafood. But don't overdo it by taking supplements: Dr. Mulrow says too much magnesium can give you a nasty case of diarrhea.

Keep up your calcium. The link between calcium intake and blood pressure is controversial. Some studies show that extra calcium can lower blood pressure, while others show that it has no effect.

But experts aren't yet convinced that large doses of calcium are going to help. Dr. Mulrow says getting the DV of 800 milligrams per day—three eight-ounce glasses of skim milk provide more than enough—and keeping your other risk factors under control is the best advice for now. Other calcium sources include low-fat cheeses, canned salmon, and other canned fish with bones. If you want to take calcium supplements, see your doctor, since too much calcium can cause other problems, such as kidney stones.

Fill up with fiber. A Swedish study of 32 people with mild high blood pressure found that taking a seven-gram tablet of fiber each day helps lower diastolic blood pressure by five points. No one is sure why; perhaps it's because of weight loss due to people being fuller and eating less, or because they eat less sodium. Whatever the reason, seven extra grams of fiber is easy to find. There's almost that much in a bowl of high-fiber cereal.

Drink in moderation. "A little alcohol isn't going to hurt," Dr. Mulrow says. "But drinking every day, and drinking to excess, could mean trouble." For women fighting high blood pressure, three ounces of alcohol a week seems to be about the limit. That means six 12-ounce beers, six 4-ounce glasses of wine, or six cocktails containing 1 ounce of hard liquor a week. (One 12-ounce beer, one 4-ounce glass of wine and one cocktail made with 1 ounce of hard liquor all have the same alcohol content of 0.5 ounce.) A 12-year study of 1,643 women, with a mean age of 47, showed that both systolic and diastolic pressure readings begin to rise steadily when the women drank any more than that.

Stop smoking. Smoking markedly increases your risk of developing a stroke or blood vessel damage from high blood pressure, says Dr. Mulrow. When you smoke, it encourages your body to deposit cholesterol within your coronary arteries. This decreases the size of your vessels and forces your heart to work harder. "Anyone with high blood pressure should stop smoking immediately," advises Dr. Mulrow.

Control Cholesterol

Experts say that by making some moderate lifestyle adjustments, you can dramatically lower your blood cholesterol level. Studies show that for every 1 percent cut in your cholesterol level, you can deflate your chances of a heart attack by 2 percent. With dietary changes alone, you can whittle away an average of 10 percent of your cholesterol reading—and perhaps even more. Margo Denke, M.D., assistant professor of medicine at the University of Texas Southwestern Medical

Center at Dallas' Center for Human Nutrition, and a member of the nutrition committee of the American Heart Association, says that the higher your cholesterol count, the greater impact a heart-healthy diet can have. For example, a woman with a cholesterol reading of 280 may be able to steamroll 25 percent off the top just by eating right.

To outmaneuver high cholesterol and the havoc it can wreak, give these cholesterol busters a try.

Switch fat. "Decreasing saturated fat is the most effective anticholesterol strategy you can use," says Karen Miller-Kovach, R.D., chief nutritionist at Weight Watchers International in Jericho, New York. That means eating less red meat, butter, cheese, whole milk, and ice cream, all of which raise LDL and total cholesterol levels. On the other hand, monounsaturated fat, known as the good fat, can actually help decrease cholesterol.

"When you switch from a diet high in saturated fat to one high in monounsaturated fat, and your weight stays about the same, your LDL cholesterol will fall while the HDL cholesterol remains stable," says Robert Rosenson, M.D., director of the Preventive Cardiology Center at Rush-Presbyterian-St. Luke's Medical Center in Chicago. "That's why olive oil is so popular, since it's high in monounsaturates." Better yet, increase your consumption of fatty fish, such as salmon and tuna. The fat in these fish are monounsaturates.

Eat less cholesterol. As important as reducing saturated fat can be, don't forget about dietary cholesterol. Any cholesterol in your blood that isn't produced by your own body comes from your diet. Here's how to keep it under control.

Try to eliminate organ meats (such as liver) from your diet. Limit the amount of lean meat, poultry, and fish to three ounces a day. And when it comes to eggs, limit your consumption of yolks to no more than two a week. Make your own cookies, cakes, and pies, and use egg whites and egg substitute when you bake or cook.

Finally, when you're going through the buffet line, reach with gusto for vegetables, fruits, and grains, which contain absolutely no dietary cholesterol. But show some willpower in holding out against high-fat salad dressings, sauces, and butter.

Feed on fiber. Fiber is just what the doctor ordered to help fill the void as saturated fat beats a retreat in your meal planning. Concentrate on soluble fiber, the kind that's jam-packed in dried beans, lentils, citrus fruits, peas, and apples. Adding soluble fiber to your diet could help lower your blood cholesterol by 5 to 10 percent.

Feel your oats. Oat bran has been on a roll for years. But how much is hype, and how much holds water? Researchers at the University of Minnesota in Minneapolis reviewed all the studies examining the power of oats and reached an artery-cleansing conclusion: Add 1 ⅓ cups of oat bran cereal (or three packets of instant oatmeal) to your daily diet, and watch your cholesterol level dip by two to three percent. If your cholesterol level is already high, you'll reap even more benefits, with oat bran skimming six to seven percent off the top.

Get fit. This one won't surprise you: Exercise does a body good. In fact, to get your HDL level high, jump into an exercise class and work up a sweat. And don't worry about having to go to extremes. "We've learned that even moderate aerobic exercise (brisk walking, jogging, swimming) raises HDLs, although this often takes six months to a year to occur," says Dr. Rosenson.

Trim your tummy. Too many women lead lives of diet desperation, with not much to show for their efforts but a lot of frustration. But a sensible, moderate weight loss program can hit your cholesterol where it hurts. Dr. Denke has found that when young women are carrying around excess body weight, their total and LDL cholesterol levels tend to be higher, and their HDL levels are lower. Losing weight produces the reverse effect.

Consider estrogen. Because natural estrogen protects you against cholesterol problems during your premenopausal years, doesn't it make sense that estrogen replacement therapy after menopause might do the same? In fact, that's exactly what research shows: Estrogen replacement therapy can cut your LDL cholesterol and raise your HDL cholesterol by about 15 percent each, according to an American Heart Association report on cardiovascular disease in women.

23

At the same time, however, estrogen replacement therapy has some red flags of its own, particularly a link to cancers of the endometrium and perhaps of the breast. You and your doctor need to keep these factors in mind when weighing the pros and cons of using estrogen replacement therapy in the war on cholesterol. Fortunately, doctors believe that by combining estrogen with progestin (another female hormone), you may be able to reduce your cancer risk.

Head off Heart Disease

Heart disease doesn't happen overnight. Most heart disease results from a narrowing of the coronary arteries, known as atherosclerosis, that takes place over decades. What makes arteries narrow? Largely, it's the way we Americans live our lives. In some other countries where lifestyles are simpler, arteries are healthy and wide open, even in the very elderly.

WHAT'S A HEALTHY WEIGHT, ANYWAY?

You don't need to be a slave to the scale. "Your healthy weight is what's produced by healthy eating and healthy exercise," says John Foreyt, Ph.D., director of the Nutritional Research Clinic at Baylor College of Medicine in Houston. "That's your goal, period."

But maybe you'd feel better with a weight range to aim for. If so, the chart below, developed by the federal government, will give you a general idea of where you should stand. These guidelines were prepared for both men and women; women will generally fall toward the lower end of each range.

HEIGHT	WEIGHT (lb.)	
	Age 19-34	Age 35 and up
5'0"	97-128	108-138
5'1"	101-132	111-143
5'2"	104-137	115-148
5'3"	107-141	119-152
5'4"	111-146	122-157
5'5"	114-150	126-162
5'6"	118-155	130-167
5'7"	121-160	134-172
5'8"	125-164	138-178
5'9"	129-169	142-183
5'10"	132-174	146-188
5'11"	136-179	151-194
6'0"	140-184	155-199
6'1"	144-189	159-205
6'2"	148-195	164-210
6'3"	152-200	168-216
6'4"	156-205	173-222
6'5"	160-211	177-228
6'6"	164-216	182-234

Many experts say that a triglyceride level above 200 milligrams per deciliter should serve as a warning flag. What's one of the best ways to temper your triglycerides? Regular exercise, says Peter Wood, Ph.D., professor of medicine emeritus and associate director of the Stanford University Center for Research in Disease Prevention in Palo Alto, California.

Maintain your best weight. In a country that seems obsessed with thinness, a lot of us could never be mistaken for being undernourished. About 19 million American women are a bit more than pleasantly plump (approximately 20 percent or more over their desirable weights). It's a little like playing Russian roulette with their hearts. In the Nurses' Health Study at Harvard Medical School, 40 percent of heart disease cases were attributed to the buildup of excess pounds.

So whether or not you consider flab to be unattractive, it's clearly hazardous to your heart. "If you're obese, the heart has to work harder to move nutrients to the additional cells in your body," says James Martin, M.D., family physician with the Institute for Urban Family Health at Beth Israel Medical Center in New York City. That extra strain on the heart can be particularly worrisome if you already have other risk factors that can contribute to heart disease, such as high cholesterol or high blood pressure. Set some goals for shedding extra pounds by relying more on low-fat foods and getting more exercise.

Sweat a little. Sure, it's tempting to toss out the exercise shoes, cancel your health club membership, and spend every weekend entrenched like Gibraltar in front of the television or camped out on the beach with a best-selling novel. If that's your idea of Shangri-la, you're not alone—but you are paying a price. In fact, almost 60 percent of American women don't get any exercise, a lifestyle choice that greatly increases their risk of heart attack.

Exercise can do more than just get you some fresh air and make you feel more invigorated. "It strengthens the heart muscle," says Dr. Wood. "With regular exercise, the heart becomes a more efficient pump. As a result, the heart rate becomes slower for a given amount of effort." Each beat is more efficient, he says, so the heart doesn't need to work as hard as it would if you were out of shape.

Exercise is particularly important if you're trying to lose weight. "When women lose weight, their HDL cholesterol levels tend to decrease," cautions Dr. Rosenson. "To maintain your HDLs at the same level or even produce a slight increase, you need to exercise while you're losing weight through diet."

Consider aspirin. It may not be the fountain of youth, but the drug that can keep your heart vital may be as close as the medicine cabinet in your bathroom. Aspirin, the tiny white pill that has been relied on a

ARE YOU AN APPLE OR A PEAR?

In the fruit basket, pears tend to age somewhat faster than apples. But when it comes to your heart—and "pear" and "apple" are describing different body shapes—the pear definitely ages slower.

Fortunately, most obese women tend to be shaped like pears (with their extra weight around their hips) rather than apples (with their fat tucked into their midsections). But that isn't always the case, particularly in women after menopause. Studies clearly show that an apple shape creates a higher risk of heart attack (as well as of diabetes, stroke, and high blood pressure).

Why is a jelly belly so malicious? One theory is that abdominal fat is more easily converted to cholesterol.

No matter what the cause turns out to be, make an effort to trim the size of your own "apple" by losing a few of those extra pounds. Here's a guideline for you to keep in mind: To cut your risk, your waist measurement should not be more than 80 percent of your hip measurement.

zillion times to zap headaches and other mild pain problems, appears to be a heart-saver as well.

In one study, over a six-year period, women who took from one to six aspirin tablets per week had about a 32 percent decreased chance of having a first heart attack compared with women who took no aspirin. Women older than age 50 seemed to get the most protection. But consult your doctor before self-prescribing aspirin, particularly if you're prone to bleeding problems, since it's a medication that discourages blood clotting in your body.

Get your vitamins. For decades, mainstream doctors have considered vitamin supplements just a small step away from quackery. Not anymore. A study published in the *New England Journal of Medicine* involving more than 87,000 women concluded that women who took vitamin E supplements for more than two years had about a 40 percent lower risk of major heart disease than those who did not take supplements.

What's the secret of vitamin E? The vitamin is an antioxidant, meaning that it protects cells from malicious molecules called free radicals that trigger a process called oxidation, which can contribute to the clogging of arteries.

"I'm giving vitamin E to my patients in standard doses that do not pose risks," says Marianne J. Legato, M.D., author of *The Female Heart* and associate professor of clinical medicine at Columbia University College of Physicians and Surgeons in New York City. Dr. Legato advises supplements of 400 international units of vitamin E, along with 1,500 milligrams of vitamin C and 6 milligrams of supplemental calcium, which studies have shown may help prevent heart disease.

Seek hormonal help. Your doctor can prescribe supplemental estrogen in your postmenopausal years, which can empower you to take a bite out of heart disease before it bites you. A Harvard University study of more than 48,000 women found that estrogen replacement therapy could slash the risk of major coronary disease and fatal cardiovascular disease by more than half.

But there's an important caveat to keep in mind: There has been concern that estrogen can increase your risk of cancer of the endometrium (the lining of the uterus) and perhaps of breast cancer. But by prescribing lower doses of estrogen and combining estrogen with progestin (the synthetic form of another hormone called progesterone), your doctor may be able to counteract these threats. You and your doctor need to weigh the pros and cons before deciding whether estrogen alone or in combination with progestin is right for you.

Breast Care
The Breast Self-Exam

Good breast care begins with learning when and how to do a breast self-exam.

Doctors agree that a self-exam should be done every month, during the first week after your period. Your goal is twofold: one, to become so familiar with the normal ridges, lumps, and bumps in your breasts that anything out of the ordinary will be very apparent, and two, to detect any lump (about a half-inch in size, for example) that suddenly appears, stays in the same place, and remains for one or two months.

What's the best way to do a self-exam? Any way you feel comfortable, doctors say. Some women prefer to do it in the shower when their breasts are slippery with soap. Others prefer to do it standing in front of a mirror. Still others prefer to do it lying on their backs.

Here's how doctors suggest you make a breast exam as accurate as possible.

Stretch first. Stretch your arms over your head and look in the mirror to see if there are any obvious changes in your breasts. Look for something major: a dimpling you've never noticed before or a nipple that has suddenly inverted, developed eczema, or has a discharge that isn't a result of being squeezed. Put your hands on your hips, push your shoulders back, and look for changes again. Then push your shoulders forward, contracting your chest muscles. Any dimpling should be obvious in this position.

Choose a search strategy. There are several different ways to do the breast exam itself: You can use the nipple as a focal point and feel for lumps along imaginary lines radiating out from the nipple all the way up to the collarbone and down to the brassiere line; you can use the nipple as a center and keep circling it with your fingers in ever-larger circles; or you can simply imagine a grid placed over your breast and examine it in up-to-the-collarbone and down-to-the-bra-line strips.

Whichever method you choose, put the hand on the side you want to examine behind your head before you start. This shifts any breast tissue that's under your armpit over to the chest wall where you can check it thoroughly.

Get into the Habit

Treat breast self-examination (BSE) like a standing appointment—mark it on your calendar. If your periods come like clockwork, simply mark "BSE" in the square a week after the day your period is scheduled to begin each month. That's the time of the menstrual cycle when your breasts should be the least painful and lumpy.

If your period is more unpredictable, or if you're postmenopausal, you may find it helpful to schedule your BSE session on the first of every month. Or link it to another monthly activity, like a standing haircut appointment.

Research suggests that having a "BSE buddy" may help, too. That means pairing up with a close friend and agreeing to remind each other with a phone call or a note when it's time for your monthly exam.

Gynecological Care
Your Best Protection

If you are on the Pill or plan to start, here's what you need to know.

See your doctor annually. Your decision to start, stay with, or get off the Pill should be based on your own health history. So you should see your doctor on an annual basis. Don't hesitate to ask questions and get her opinion. Don't be afraid to seek a second opinion. Remember that a lot of doctors feel that the benefits generally outweigh the risks for healthy, nonsmoking women.

Know your family history. If anyone in your family has had heart disease, breast cancer, high blood pressure, ovarian cancer, or uterine cancer, discuss it with your doctor. These factors should be taken into consideration, but they won't immediately prohibit you from taking

28

BREAST SELF-EXAM (BSE)

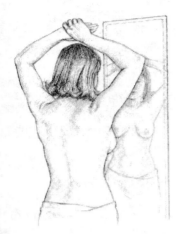

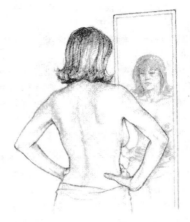

Put your arms over your head and look for any dimpling, nipple discharge, or other changes in appearance.

Put your hands on your hips, push your shoulders first back, then forward, and look for any changes in your breasts.

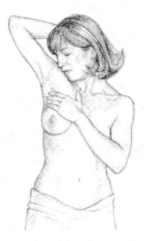

Place your right hand behind your head. With the finger pads of your left hand, examine your entire right breast from collarbone to bra line and into your armpit. Repeat the process on your left breast with your left hand behind your head. See the opposite page for a description of the different search strategies.

the Pill, says Edward Linn, M.D., chairman of obstetrics and gynecology at Lutheran General Hospital in Park Ridge, Illinois.

Protect yourself. The Pill may protect you from pregnancy, but it won't protect you from sexually transmitted diseases or AIDS. One answer is condoms. Latex condoms containing the spermicide nonoxynol-9 are most effective against sexually transmitted diseases, experts say.

Practice prevention. Performing a monthly breast self-examination is always important, but if you're on the Pill, make certain you do it routinely. Doctors also recommend that you have your first mammogram between the ages of 35 and 40, then one every two years during your forties and one every year thereafter.

How to Assure Pap Accuracy

The Pap is a snap—a simple procedure in which your doctor scrapes cells from your cervix and smears them onto a glass slide. The slide is sent to a laboratory, where the sample cells are dyed (so they are more visible) and examined under a microscope by specially trained laboratory personnel known as cytotechnologists. Abnormal samples are sent to a pathologist for confirmation.

Theoretically, the Pap test should detect any abnormal cervical cells. But the American College of Obstetricians and Gynecologists estimates that 15 to 40 percent of Pap smears are reported "normal" when in fact cell abnormalities are present. Poor cell-sampling techniques, hard-to-read slides, or a bad call by an overburdened screener is usually to blame.

For better Pap results:

☐ Abstain from sexual intercourse for 12 hours before a test. Semen can interfere with test results. And sometimes sex can cause microscopic vaginal tears.

☐ Schedule the Pap smear in the middle of your menstrual cycle. The exact timing isn't critical, but you should avoid the days of your menstrual period, since blood can obscure cells on the slide.

☐ Postpone your Pap test if you have an active yeast infection. Inflammation from the infection can mask dysplastic cells on your cervix.

☐ Don't douche or wear a tampon for at least 72 hours before the test. You may reduce the number of cells available for examination.

☐ Ask your doctor if she uses both a cytology brush and a spatula for cell collection. The two used in combination detect more cellular abnormalities than any other method or either alone. The cytology brush looks like a pipe cleaner and is more efficient than a cotton swab or wooden spatula for sampling cells inside the cervix (the transformation zone), where 95 percent of cervical cancers start. The wooden spatula is still the best tool for sampling cells on the outside of the cervix.

☐ Call your gynecologist for your Pap test results in about a week. Don't assume that all is well if you don't hear from your doctor: Your paperwork could have slipped through the cracks. Ask for a copy of the written report to keep for your own records.

☐ If you need to repeat the test, don't schedule it right away. If the surface of the cervix is rescraped within six weeks, the follow-up smear has a 60 percent chance of being a false normal. The first Pap may have removed the few abnormal cells; after a few months, a second test can better tell if they have grown back.

Cancer Prevention

Some cancers can take more than 30 years to develop. So what you do now can have a tremendous impact on your ability to have a long, healthy, and cancer-free life, says John Laszlo, M.D., national vice-president for research at the American Cancer Society. In fact, oncologists estimate that perhaps 50 percent of cancers could be prevented if women made just a few simple adjustments in their lifestyles. Here's where to start.

Become an ex-smoker. Smokers are 10 times more likely to develop lung cancer, and up to 30 percent of all cancer deaths are caused by smoking, says Earnest Rosenbaum, M.D., an oncologist at the University of California, San Francisco/Mount Zion and author of *You Can Prevent Cancer*. Studies also suggest that women who smoke are twice as likely to get cervical cancer. So if you don't smoke, don't start, and if you smoke, quit.

Watch out for passive smoke. Up to 8,000 lung cancer deaths a year among nonsmokers can be attributed to secondhand smoke, says Charles B. Simone, M.D., an oncologist in Princeton, New Jersey, and author of *Cancer and Nutrition*. If people in your household smoke, ask them to quit, or establish an area where they can smoke without endangering you.

Fill up on fiber. Women who eat lots of fibrous fruits, vegetables, and whole grains, such as broccoli, brussels sprouts, cabbage, apples, bananas, mangoes, and whole-wheat cereals and breads, may have fewer breast, colon, and rectal cancers than those who don't eat these foods, Dr. Simone says. Fiber reduces the amount of estrogen in the blood. Estrogen may alter cell structure and promotes breast cancer, says Carl Mansfield, M.D., professor and chairman of the Department of Radiation Oncology and Nuclear Medicine at Thomas Jefferson University Hospital in Philadelphia. In addition, fiber helps speed stool

31

through your body and reduce exposure of your digestive tract to carcinogens.

Fiber also may help prevent other cancers. In a study of 399 women with endometrial cancer and 296 disease-free women, Louise Brinton, Ph.D., chief of the Environmental Studies Section at the National Cancer Institute in Rockville, Maryland, found that women who ate more than two daily servings of high-fiber breads and cereals had a 40 percent lower risk of developing endometrial cancer.

The National Cancer Institute recommends that women eat at least 20 to 30 grams of fiber a day. If you start your day with a cereal that has at least 7 grams of fiber per serving, add another 3 grams of fiber by topping your cereal with one medium sliced banana and two tablespoons of raisins. Then you're halfway to the minimum daily recommendation, says Gladys Block, Ph.D., professor of public health nutrition at the University of California in Berkeley. Then all you need to do is make sure you get three more servings of fruits, vegetables, and/or grains through the rest of the day. Beans, for example, are particularly high in fiber.

Go for vegetables. Eat at least five servings of fruits and vegetables a day, Dr. Rosenbaum says. These foods contain antioxidant vitamins and minerals such as beta-carotene, selenium, and vitamins A and E that combat the formation of cancer-causing free radicals.

Take a supplement. Supplements containing vitamins C and E and other antioxidant vitamins and minerals can help neutralize certain carcinogens such as the nitrites found in bacon, sausage, hot dogs, and cured meats, according to Kedar N. Prasad, Ph.D., director of the Center for Vitamins and Cancer Research at the University of Colorado Health Sciences Center in Denver and author of *Vitamins in Cancer Prevention and Treatment*. Supplements also can strengthen your body's immune system so that it can destroy newly formed cancer cells before they multiply, Dr. Prasad says. He suggests taking 15 milligrams of beta-carotene once a day, 2,500 international units of vitamin A twice a day, 500 milligrams of vitamin C twice a day, 200 milligrams (or 134 international units) of vitamin E twice a day, and 50 micrograms of selenium twice a day.

Trim the fat. The high-fat diet many American women eat is believed to trigger cancer. Researchers at the University of Hawaii at Manoa compared the fat consumption of 272 postmenopausal women who had breast cancer with that of 296 women who were cancer-free. The researchers found a significant association between breast cancer and eating sausage, processed cold cuts, beef, and lamb.

Throw away the deep fryer. Frying simply adds more fat to food, and fat promotes cancer. Broil, steam, bake, or boil your food instead, Dr.

SEVEN SIGNS YOU SHOULDN'T IGNORE

Here are seven common warning signs of cancer. If you develop any of them, contact your doctor immediately.

1. A lump or thickening in the breast.
2. A change in a wart or a mole.
3. A sore that doesn't heal.
4. A change in bowel or bladder habits.
5. A persistent cough or hoarseness.
6. Constant indigestion or trouble swallowing.
7. Unusual bleeding or discharge.

Mansfield says. Brown or sauté in nonstick pans, or use vegetable spray or chicken broth.

Go easy on the barbecue. The smoke and heat of charbroiling creates several cancer-causing substances, including nitrosamine, one of the most potent carcinogens known, Dr. Mansfield says. If you like to barbecue, do it carefully and sparingly, Dr. Prasad suggests. Place the grill as far above the coals as possible, and wrap aluminum foil around the grill to prevent fat from dripping onto the flame and causing excessive smoke and charring.

Lose weight. If you're overweight, you could be producing more estrogen than you need. Excessive amounts of estrogen have been linked to increased risk of breast cancer, Dr. Mansfield says. Keep your weight within the range suggested by your gynecologist or family physician.

Don't douche too often. Researchers at the Uniformed Services University of the Health Sciences in Bethesda, Maryland, found that cervical cancer risk was four to five times higher in women who douched more than four times a month. Women who douched less had no increased risk. The type of douching liquid made little difference in risk. The researchers speculate that too-frequent cleansing may upset the cervix's normal chemical balance, diluting secretions or destroying friendly bacteria that may protect against viral invaders.

Practice safe sex. Human papilloma virus (HPV), a sexually transmitted disease, has been linked to precancerous changes in the cervix called dysplasia. Multiple sex partners and unprotected sex are the two major risk factors for HPV. Use condoms and maintain a mutually monogamous relationship, Dr. Rosenbaum suggests.

33

Check out your family tree. Although less than 10 percent of cancers have genetic roots, finding out if cancer runs in your family can help your doctor evaluate your risk and recommend ways to prevent the disease or detect it early, Dr. Rosenbaum says. Include as many relatives on both sides of your family as you can. If someone had cancer, jot down the age at which they were diagnosed and the organ in which it originated.

Focus on high-folate foods. At this point, it's a little early to say anything certain about folate's role in cervical cancer. But it's not too early to adopt a prudent stance with regard to your folate intake, especially if you smoke, take oral contraceptives, or are pregnant. "The problem is, we find that many individuals are either taking in very small amounts of folate or have a low-folate status," says Howard E. Sauberlich, Ph.D., a professor in the Department of Nutrition at the University of Alabama in Birmingham.

Folate is widely available in dark leafy green vegetables, legumes, fruits, and certain grains. Some sources include beans (½ cup has 130 micrograms), cooked spinach (½ cup has 130 micrograms), orange juice (1 cup has 110 micrograms), and wheat germ (1 ounce has 100 micrograms).

Bone Health

34

Healthy Habits for Life and Limb

Doctors agree that women at the greatest risk for osteoporosis are those with family histories of the disease or personal histories of smoking or heavy drinking. If you have a higher than normal level of bone loss, don't despair—it's probably not too late to start building bone.

Here are the best ways to strengthen your skeleton.

Pump up your calcium. Calcium is to your bones what air is to your lungs—the element they need to be healthy. Ninety-nine percent of the calcium in your diet goes straight to your bones. If you don't get enough calcium, you can't make enough bone—it's as simple as that.

Although the DV for women is 800 milligrams a day, you need more calcium in adolescence and after menopause, says Clifford Rosen, M.D., director of the Maine Center for Osteoporosis Research and Education in Bangor. Women should get at least 1,000 milligrams before menopause and 1,500 milligrams after menopause. Although food is the best way to get calcium, what matters most is that you take in the recommended amount, says Dr. Rosen. If that's through food, fine; if it's through a combination of food and calcium supplements, fine. Just make sure the numbers add up.

Ounce for ounce, milk and milk products are the best sources of dietary calcium. One eight-ounce serving of nonfat yogurt provides about

450 milligrams of calcium. One cup of skim milk offers more than 300 milligrams. Many other foods contain calcium, but the nutrient isn't as easily absorbed from these foods as it is from dairy products.

Don't forget the D. Bones don't absorb calcium unless they have plenty of vitamin D, says Michael F. Holick, M.D., Ph.D., director of the Vitamin D, Skin and Bone Research Laboratory at Boston University Medical Center. Without vitamin D, your body absorbs about 10 percent of the calcium it takes in; with vitamin D, it can absorb 80 to 90 percent. "Vitamin D tells the small intestine, 'Here comes the calcium. Open up and let it in,'" explains Dr. Holick. The DV for vitamin D is five micrograms or 200 international units—easily found in fortified foods such as milk, breads, and cereals.

Besides getting some of your daily vitamin D through food, your body can make it from sunshine, which triggers a vitamin D manufacturing process in your skin. Just 5 to 15 minutes of bright sunshine every day, before you apply sunscreen, will supply your needs, says Dr. Rosen. If you live north of New York City, however, you can't depend on the sun. In that case, you'll need to be sure you're getting enough vitamin D from dietary sources. (If you're getting plenty in your diet, you won't need time in the sun at all.)

Review your medications. Certain medications—thyroid medications; anti-inflammatory steroids such as hydrocortisone (Locoid), cortisone (Cortone Acetate), and prednisone (Key-Pred 50); anticonvulsants such as phenytoin (Dilantin); depressants such as phenobarbital (Barbita); and the diuretic furosemide (Lasix)—can cause osteoporosis, particularly when they're taken regularly in high doses over a number of years. Thyroid medications in normal doses should pose no problem, however, says Dr. Rosen, and the risk from diuretics can be offset by taking additional calcium. The most serious osteoporosis risk is from steroids, Dr. Rosen says. If you require long-term steroid medication, your doctor may recommend additional anti-osteoporosis medications such as calcitonin (Cibacalcin) or hormone replacement therapy in addition to calcium and vitamin D supplements, he says.

Keep 'em dry and healthy. "Alcohol actually poisons the cells that build bone," says Susan Allen, M.D., Ph.D., assistant professor of internal medicine at the University of Missouri-Columbia School of Medicine. A beer or glass of wine now and then probably won't cause you much harm. But avoid drinking to excess, she says—more than two to three drinks a day.

Don't puff. Smoking lowers your levels of estrogen, says Barbara S. Levine, Ph.D., associate clinical professor of nutrition in medicine and director of the Calcium Information Center at Cornell University

Medical College in New York City. And lower estrogen, she says, means less protection against bone loss.

Consider hormone replacement therapy. For some women past menopause, hormone replacement therapy can thicken bones. Ask your doctor whether you're a candidate for it.

Enjoy weight-bearing exercise. To strengthen bones, you need activities in which you're bearing weight on your bones, says Gail Dalsky, Ph.D., director of the Exercise Research Laboratory at the University of Connecticut Health Center in Farmington. Weight-bearing exercises include brisk walking, jogging, and dancing, which actually stimulate bone cells to build more bone, particularly in your back and hips, where you most need it, Dr. Allen says.

Pumping iron is another ideal way to build bone strength, because it increases the weight of gravity on your bones. It's good sense to make weight-lifting part of your weight-bearing exercise. Any lifting done in a standing position is particularly helpful for the spine and hips. If you've never used weights before, be sure to get your doctor's clearance and a trainer's advice on the safest routine.

Once you've found the weight-bearing exercises you like, keep at them for 30 minutes to one hour three to four times a week, Dr. Allen says.

AIDS Prevention
AIDS: Fighting the Scourge

Many of us know at least one person who has AIDS or has died from it. That's not too surprising when you consider that more than one million Americans have this fatal viral disease. But behind the grim numbers, there is a faint glimmer of hope.

"In the beginning, people were dying within months of their diagnoses. But we've learned so much more about the disease since then, and we now have long-term survivors who are very healthy for good periods of time," says Peggy Clarke, president of the American Social Health Association in Research Triangle Park, North Carolina.

Antiviral drugs such as zidovudine (AZT), didanosine (Videx), and zalcitabine (Hivid) can slow the progress of the disease, which gradually destroys the immune system, allowing life-threatening infections and cancers to invade the body at will.

But there is no cure for this deadly disease. So the best way to fight AIDS is to not get it in the first place. That means using a latex condom or having sex in a monogamous relationship in which both partners have been tested and found to be free of the human immunodeficiency virus (HIV) that causes AIDS. If you use intravenous drugs, don't share needles with others, as HIV may be transmitted through bodily fluids that remain in the needle.

WHAT'S YOUR RISK?

It's not difficult to evaluate your risk of developing osteoporosis, says Susan Allen, M.D., Ph.D., assistant professor of
internal medicine at the University of Missouri-Columbia
School of Medicine. Start with the following questions:

- Do you have a small, thin frame, or are you
  Caucasian or Asian?
- Do you have relatives with osteoporosis?
- Have you reached menopause?
- Have you had an early or surgically induced
  menopause?
- Do you take high doses of thyroid medication or corti-
  sone-like drugs for asthma, arthritis, or cancer?
- Do you avoid eating many dairy products and other
  sources of calcium?
- Are you not getting regular weight-bearing exercise
  such as brisk walking?
- Do you smoke cigarettes or drink alcohol heavily?

If you answered yes to two or more of these questions,
your risk for developing osteoporosis is high, Dr. Allen says.
It's time to talk to your doctor about developing a lifelong
prevention plan.

Before You Hit-the-Pillow Talk

The most important thing to remember when you begin a sexual relationship is that you're not crawling into bed with one man, says
Jacqueline Darroch Forrest, Ph.D., of the Alan Guttmacher Institute in
New York City. You're also sharing space with all the people *he* had sex
with—and all the people *they* had sex with!

"Our biggest problem is not contraceptive technology—the hard-
ware, so to speak—but the software of our own behavior and how we
deal with our relationships with one another," says Dr. Forrest. It's
often a lot easier to have sex than it is to talk about it.

But talk you must. And the International Planned Parenthood
Federation offers the following suggested responses for women negoti-
ating over condom use.

HE: I know I don't have any disease. I haven't had sex for a long time.

YOU: As far as I know, I don't have any disease either. But I still want us to use a condom since either of us could have an infection and not know about it.

Or:

HE: What an insult! You think I'm the sort of person who gets AIDS?

YOU: I didn't say that. Anyone can get an infection. I want to use a condom to protect us both.

Or:

HE: I love you. Would I give you an infection?

YOU: Not deliberately. But most people don't know they are infected. That's why this is best for both of us.

Other suggestions:

- Discuss condom use before you're physically close, when you can still control your feelings.
- Rehearse what you want to say to your partner. Have a close friend role-play with you.
- Bring up the subject by mentioning a news item or TV program you've seen about condoms.
- If your partner doesn't have a condom, pull one (make sure you have one at all times) out of your handbag and say something simple and clear such as, "Let's use this condom for protection."
- Be assertive. Be clear. Don't get drawn into an argument. It's your life and health at stake.

38

OPEN WIDE, REST ASSURED

Epidemologists at the Centers for Disease Control and Prevention in Atlanta studied the patients of a dentist who had AIDS, and found no evidence that he had transmitted the virus to any patients, even though he hadn't always used proper infection-control procedures. The American Dental Association offers a free brochure, "Talking Infection Control," that suggests questions for your dentist. Send a self-addressed stamped envelope to ADA Cares, Suite 930, 332 South Michigan Avenue, Chicago, IL 60604.

CHAPTER 4
YOUR HEALTH
PLANNER

A re you the kind of person who thinks you had a Pap test a year ago, but when you check, you find out it was back in 1989? That's why it's a good idea to start a notebook in which you list every major screening test you've had or might need. (See "Chapter 2: The Top 15 Tests for Women.") You can use the pages that follow to help you keep track of your doctor visits, test results, and treatments.

39

QUICK REFERENCE GUIDE: IMPORTANT PHONE NUMBERS

Use the space here to list your doctors and other practitioners. This will eliminate the need to flip through the telephone directory to find their numbers.

Doctors and Other Practitioners	Specialty	Telephone

Pharmacy	Address	Telephone

Hospital	Address	Telephone

BLOOD PRESSURE\CHOLESTEROL LEVELS\WEIGHT RECORD

Keeping track of your blood pressure, cholesterol levels, and weight is a very important part of your health plan. It's relatively easy to monitor your blood pressure and weight because blood-pressure cuffs and scales are readily available. However, cholesterol screenings require an order from your doctor and a trip to a laboratory.

Use the pages here to record your blood pressure, cholesterol levels, and weight each time you have them checked—by a medical technician or your own readings.

Date	Weight	Blood Pressure	Cholesterol		
			LDL	HDL	Total

DOCTOR VISIT RECORDS

Use the space here to record your visits to your doctors. This will help you keep track of your screenings and treatments.

Date	Practitioner Seen	Symptoms/ Complaints	Tests Performed	Diagnosis and Treatment

42

MEDICATIONS RECORD

Use the space here to keep track of any medications your physician has prescribed or that you have purchased over the counter. You should discuss any medications you're taking with your doctor at every visit.

Date Purchased/ Filled	Medication/ Product	Prescribing Physician	Exp. Date of Medicine	Pharmacy Where Filled	Side Effects/ Adverse Reactions

43

ROUTINE SCREENINGS

Below are the top 15 tests for women as recommended in Chapter 2. Next to each, list the date on which it was performed and the results. Also, note when you should schedule a follow-up screening.

Test	Date	Results	Schedule Follow-up
Blood Pressure Check			
Blood Cholesterol Check			
Exercise Stress Test			
Breast Self-Examination			
Breast Exam by a Physician			
Mammography			
Pelvic Examination			
Pap Test			
Transvaginal Ultrasound			
Endometrial Tissue Sample			
Digital-Rectal Exam			
Fecal Occult Blood Test			
Sigmoidoscopy			
Bone Scan			
HIV Test			

ADDITIONAL NOTES

_____

_____

_____

_____

_____

_____

_____

_____

_____

_____

_____

_____

_____

_____

ADDITIONAL NOTES

_____

_____

_____

_____

_____

_____

_____

_____

_____

_____

_____

_____

_____

_____

We'd like to hear from you. Please let us know
what you liked about this book. Write:

101 Female Health Secrets Every Woman Must Know
c/o Project Editor
33 East Minor Street
Emmaus, PA 18098

Rodale Press also publishes the following health books:

New Choices in Natural Healing - Over 1,000 of the best self-help remedies from the world of alternative medicine.

Total Health for Women - From allergies and back pain to overweight and PMS, the best preventive and curative advice for 110 women's health problems.

Total Health for Men - How to prevent and treat the health problems that trouble men most.

The Complete Book of Natural and Medicinal Cures - How to choose the most potent healing agents for over 200 conditions and diseases.

Curing Fatigue - A step-by-step plan to uncover and eliminate the causes of chronic fatigue.

Disease Free - How to prevent, treat and cure more than 150 illnesses and conditions.

The Doctors Book of Home Remedies - Thousands of tips and techniques anyone can use to heal everyday health problems.

The Doctors Book of Home Remedies for Children - From allergies and animal bites to toothaches and TV addiction, hundreds of doctor-proven techniques and tips to care for your kid.

The Healthy Woman - Delivers up-to-the-minute information on everything from woman's health to fashion trends, from medical insights about sexuality to the latest in skin care.

To place an order, call 1-800-527-8200.